THE STORY OF HOLYWELL HOSPITAL:
A COUNTRY ASYLUM

Antrim's Holywell Hospital was opened as an asylum
'98 there have been great changes in the treatment of
l illness and the way it is viewed in society. In the past
vell was often overcrowded and underfunded. There were
mics of infectious diseases and, in 1930, a devastating
hen, particularly under Dr Boyd's leadership, great
were made to inject energy into the social life of
ts and staff, and to make the hospital an increasingly
nt place to be. Instead of being restrained and forgotten,
entally ill are given hope and are rightly able to feel they
valued part of society.

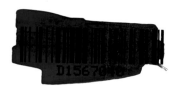

By the same author:

Ulster & Its Future After the Troubles (1977)
Ulster & The German Solution (1978)
Ulster & The British Connection (1979)
Ulster & The Lords of the North (1980)
Ulster & The Middle Ages (1982)
Ulster & St Patrick (1984)
The Twilight Pagans (1990)
Enemy of England (1991)
The Great Siege (2002)
Ulster in the Age of Saint Comgall of Bangor (2004)
Ulster Blood (2005)
King William's Victory (2006)
Ulster Stock (2007)
Famine in the Land of Ulster (2008)
Pre-Christian Ulster (2009)
The Glens of Antrim (2010)
Ulster Women – A Short History (2010)
The Invasion of Ulster (2010)
Ulster in the Viking Age (2011)
Ulster in the Eighteenth Century (2011)
Ulster in the History of Ireland (2012)
Rathlin Island (2013)
Saint Patrick's Missionary Journeys in Ireland (2015)
The Story of Carrickfergus (2015)
Ireland's Holy Places (2016)
The Conqueror of the North (2017)

THE STORY OF HOLYWELL HOSPITAL: A COUNTRY ASYLUM

Michael Sheane

ARTHUR H. STOCKWELL LTD
Torrs Park, Ilfracombe, Devon, EX34 8BA
Established 1898
www.ahstockwell.co.uk

Dedication: To the staff and patients of Holywell Hospital, Antrim.

ISBN 978-0-7223-4856-7
Printed in Great Britain by
Arthur H. Stockwell Ltd
Torrs Park   Ilfracombe
Devon EX34 8BA

CONTENTS

Chapter One   *A Fit Place to Build an Asylum*   7

Chapter Two   *The Formation Years: 1898–1932*   13

Chapter Three *New Horizons: 1932–47*   19

Chapter Four   *A National Health Service Hospital*   26

CHAPTER ONE

A FIT PLACE TO BUILD AN ASYLUM

The need to build a new asylum was due to overcrowding in the Belfast institution. In 1847 Belfast Asylum contained 252 patients. The male wards were overcrowded and the female wards were close to capacity. This did not bode well for the morale of the patients. In 1891 a site of some 100 acres at Holywell, Antrim, was chosen for the new hospital. The grounds lay about two miles away on the north side of the town, on high ground and commanding a view of Lough Neagh. Eventually Holywell and its farms were to cover 411 acres. The site of the hospital may have been the site of a monastery in the fifth century, with its long association with the famous round tower, known as the Steeple.

The board of governors met for the first time on 31 January 1893. They decided upon the basic structure of the proposed asylum. There were to be two hospital pavilions for acute cases to contain eighty males and eighty females respectively; also two other pavilions to contain 100 males and 100 females respectively. There was also to be an administration block to provide accommodation for 500 patients and to include kitchen, laundry, stores, workshops, and a dining hall to house 300 patients. There was to be a church, open to both Protestants and Catholics; there was also to be a mortuary. Holywell House was to be the residence for the medical superintendent.

The new asylum would cost £58,794, but its construction was fraught with difficulties. The hospital was due to be opened in 1896, but a later date was more likely – August 1897. The hospital was opened in 1898 and consisted of two long corridors running from a clock tower and reception area. Various buildings, wards, offices, halls and so on branched off these corridors. Around Holywell were high walls enclosing the buildings, and an 'airing court' where patients would be able to have outdoor exercise.

In May 1898, in readiness to receive the first patients, Dr Samuel Graham was appointed resident medical superintendent. Until the new building was completed patients could be treated in the forecourt of the recently purchased Spring Farm House. By the end of 1898 thirty-two male patients were transferred from Belfast Asylum to Spring Farm House. By the end of 1898 eighty-four males and 101 females had been transferred from Belfast. It was observed that there were no escapes during this period. In January 1898 a special meeting was called with the Board of Control to discuss the great delay in the completion of Holywell. Also, the boiler and electrical supply were behind schedule, so now the relevant penalties were invoked. On 27 March 1899 the thirty-two patients accommodated in Spring Farm House were at last moved into the chronic block of the main building. Holywell's governors said that unless the contract was completed the contractors would be changed. They demanded another £6,500 for extra work, but the board of governors refused and said the contractors would be taken to court. The board of governors entered first into legal arbitration, and a settlement was wanted out of court. The board itself agreed to pay Messrs Martin an extra £2,000. Lanyon, the architect of the hospital, died in 1900.

The clock tower was topped with gleaming copper, which reflected the sunlight across the countryside, while the clock itself was illuminated at night. It provided a beacon for boats on Lough Neagh, guiding boats into the Six Mile Water and from there to Antrim town. The hospital was a classic Victorian asylum; it was a testament to the middle-class culture of the age. By 1900 all patients from Belfast Asylum had been admitted to Holywell, and the first direct admissions were accepted. For the first years of care the patients were plagued by teething problems. The chronic block – both male and female – was fully occupied. But there had been no cases of violence. A large number of male patients were employed on the farm, giving rise to good physical health for the patients, and leading to an improvement in mental health. The female patients were employed in the wards in sewing and knitting. All patients were encouraged to spend some time in the fresh air. But the recreation hall had not yet been completed, so there were no patient amusements available. There were regular religious services for Presbyterians, Anglicans and Roman Catholics. A small number of newspapers and magazines were provided, and a few patients were employed in the workshops. Patients and staff did most of the labouring on the farm and estate. Within a few years of opening, the farm had been drained and levelled; five acres for a sewage farm had been allocated, along with seven acres for shrubs; two and a half miles of walkways were constructed, six feet across.

At first there was plenty of room in Holywell for the mentally ill, in contrast to the Belfast Asylum. The inspector of lunatics said that there was plenty of dayroom accommodation. But by 1902 there were 500 patients held – sixty in excess of capacity – and the male side was especially congested. Soon the government was pushing for an extension in accommodation and was threatening financial penalties. But in August 1905 a female patient hanged herself, and an inquiry ensued. After this the rather run-down Spring Farm House was renovated. It served as a dormitory for thirty-six patients and three staff, all of whom worked on the farm. But by the end of 1905 overcrowding was everywhere apparent; the dormitories on the male side were so overcrowded with beds that there was barely room to pass between them. The board of guardians in 1905 appointed a committee to consider increases in accommodation. Holywell was so overcrowded by 1906 that the committee decided to build a detached villa to hold seventy-four patients. The villa was to be two-storeyed, containing on the ground floor essential accommodation – i.e. two small dormitories, visiting rooms, a kitchen and the usual sanitary annexes. A covered veranda would run in the front, nearly the full length of the building. The upper floor would consist entirely of dormitories with bathing facilities and an attendant's room. The walls were built of brick, the roof tiled and window sashes made of steel. The cost was £5,250 to be repaid in instalments every six months over forty years. But the villa construction was also behind time; it shot over budget and deadline. In the contract 151 days had been allowed. In fact it took another 151 days on top of this. The board allowed fifty-one days due to severe weather conditions, but fined the constructors £1 a day for the remaining 100.

The new villa was opened in 1907; this had ended Holywell's basic constructions at a cost of £120,000, all this amount being borrowed from the commissioners of public works, and all to be repaid by County Antrim's ratepayers. However, the cost of Holywell's basic amenities, like water, sewage and heating, was also fraught with difficulty.

When it opened, Holywell's consumption of coal was about seven tons per day, so the heaviest cost was coal, the consumption of which was £2,000 plus, rising to £3,000 when the asylum was fully occupied. In time the central-heating system was abandoned altogether and replaced with open fires in the wards and rooms. The entire hospital was almost fully without heat for three decades, with adverse effects on the patients and staff. When Dr Boyd became

RMS in 1932 he was shocked at the state of heating in Holywell. In 1933 it was decided to install a new central-heating system at a cost of £6,000. Central heating was reintroduced into Holywell in 1934, so matters were made more comfortable. The hospital was now heated to a high standard. The villa and Spring Farm House were provided with central heating in 1932.

In the early 1930s the sewage system of Holywell was overhauled. The original system had become dilapidated and inefficient; the effluent was foul and concentrated. New pipes were introduced and three modern beds with revolving distributors were introduced with positive results. The cost was £1,200; the work was completed by February 1935. There was a colitis outbreak in 1937, but in 1949 it was decided to abandon Holywell's sewage system, and link it to that of Antrim Rural District Council, which took some time. It was reported in 1952 that Holywell's sewage pipes were not capable of coping with the volume of sewage passing through.

The water supply to Holywell was another problem. At first it was hoped to use the holy well itself. It was calculated that it was capable of yielding sixty gallons per minute or 86,400 gallons per day. In July 1898 it yielded 3,692 gallons per hour, or an excess of 690 gallons of that required. In May 1898 it was reported that with sufficient filtration it would be suitable for domestic use. To help matters, Lanyon proposed sinking a well at the nearby site of Ladyhill, but this had to be abandoned for the landlords feared that abstraction of water from the land would allow his tenants to gain a rent reduction. It was proposed to sink wells on the Holywell site; at a depth of 190 feet the spring seemed promising, but the scheme came to grief so attention was again drawn to the supply from the holy well, so that Holywell would have a sufficient amount of water.

By 1904 a good supply of water from a reservoir on the hill overlooking Holywell was in line with a catchment area three or four miles to the north-west of the hospital. This was supplemented with rain drawn off the roofs of the institution. There was an outbreak of typhoid fever in the asylum so that one could not drink the water supply. The Tobernaveen Well was temporarily brought back into use. Hitherto in Holywell there had been a shortage of water in the summer months. In 1937 a sample of Holywell's water was sent to Queen's University for examination, and the supply was found to be suspect. As a result several changes had to be made. At a cost of £2,500 a mechanical filtration and sterilizing plant was completed and in use. The colour of the water was noticeable.

CHAPTER TWO

THE FORMATIVE YEARS: 1898–1932

Holywell opened in 1898; there was the appointing of a board of governors in its first years of operation. Governors were mostly appointed from the great and good; they took a more direct control over the asylum. Only those who paid rates had the vote. During the twentieth century the arrangement was that only local ratepayers dealt with the problem of water supply. With Antrim booming, this Victorian ideal seemed realizable. In the twentieth century inflation and rising expectations rendered this increasingly inadequate. From 1921 to 1942 Northern Ireland struggled with unemployment, which at times was as high as twenty-five per cent. In 1874 a grant to the governors of the asylum was fixed at four shillings per patient, to lighten the burden on the local ratepayers at a time when there was an increase of patients in the hospital. The four shillings per patient was to be increased to five shillings per head. The patient population at Holywell quickly rose from 203 in 1899 to 567 in 1905. Patient numbers rose sharply, by fifty-seven to 624 in 1908. The dining hall in the hospital had become overcrowded. By 1910 the number of patients had plateaued. In 1909 there were 586; in 1910 there were 586; and in 1914 there were 588. The standard of care in the workhouse was not as good as in Holywell. Patients were admitted for a variety of reasons – often to physically protect themselves or others. One female patient from Church Street, Antrim, was admitted in January 1903 because she had no one to take care of her; she had filthy habits and was feared by the local people.

The First World War had little impact on the hospital, but the Troubles in Northern Ireland had some effect. Costs per patient in the early years of the twentieth century were about £20 per year – below the average for Irish asylums. The figure reached £57 in 1920; during the twenties it reached between £35 and £40. Up until 1921 the grant from central government varied around £5,000. Holywell headed a deputation for all the asylums in Northern Ireland, and a resolution was passed calling for the payment of arrears of the central-government grant. A payment of sixty per cent of the actual cost of maintaining the pauper asylums was made.

In 1923 the grant was fixed at £5,149; this remained in force until the Second World War. Financial conditions, however, remained stringent. The staff at Holywell included a medical superintendent, clerk, storekeeper, land steward, matron, engineers and three chaplains. The work appears not to have been highly paid. The salary for the RMS was £450 per year, plus £150 for food and lodgings, etc. However, women were discriminated against. The main problem was that of underpay.

In 1905 on the male side there were four nurses and sixteen ordinary attendants on night duty. There were also two attendants on night duty on the female side. There was neither a head nurse nor a head attendant. By 1908 there were on the male side only five charge and seventeen ordinary attendants, and on the female side only two charge and fourteen ordinary attendants. In 1909 a head nurse was finally appointed, but no staff held the Standard Royal Medico-Psychologist certificate in connection with nursing.

By 1928 there was a shortage of staff and none had

received specialist training. Working hours for staff were long. When staff entered the hospital they were faced with long hours ahead of them. The morning started at 6.30 a.m. and lasted until 7.15 p.m.; twenty minutes was allotted for breakfast, forty minutes for dinner and twenty minutes for tea. The working week lasted for about seventy hours. Male attendants were allowed to sleep out if they preferred; many did, but few staff enjoyed this privilege. Male staff had a uniform – or rather a suit of clothes normally worn on or off duty. These clothes were made in the asylum by the patients and paid for out of staff wages. Female staff only wore their uniform on duty. There were great demands put on staff in these years. Relations with the doctors were more distant – staff had to stand to attention when the doctors passed through the wards. All nurses and female attendants had to sleep in the hospital, to be near the patients. The noise from patients was always audible. Nurses were not permitted to leave the hospital grounds even after duty hours without special permission from the superintendent. These restrictions were made necessary by the small number of night staff in these early years. Some of the night staff needed backup – for example, to deal with a troublesome patient. But the possibility of fire was the main reason why the staff had to be vigilant in the hospital.

Segregation between the sexes was strict; male and female staff only mixed on special occasions, at dances, at occasional dinners and at Christmas. The RMS was a powerful figure in the hospital and in local society and enjoyed a large house in the grounds. On the wards the matron and the chief male attendant ruled with a rod of iron. Pay was poor and conditions were harsh; in 1904 a stoker lost his arm in a work accident and was laid off without compensation.

During the Great War of 1914–18 inflation resulted in regular wage claims for the staff, usually met by concessions. In July 1916 the entire staff was granted a ten-per-cent bonus pay rise. Conditions of service were at least as pressing a matter as that of wages. Employees pressed for shorter hours – no more than sixty-four hours per week. But in 1920 staff demands for higher wages and shorter working hours were turned down. Many of the staff were members of the amalgamated Transport and General Workers Union in the 1930s.

We come now to the plight of patients in Holywell.

William Nicholl, sixteen years old at the time, was among the first of the admissions in 1898. He spent his whole adult life in the hospital, for he was violent on occasions. He had broken windows in St Patrick's Boys' House on the Falls Road, so he was transferred to the new hospital.

Due to the complexities of the law, the simplest methods of admission were by juridical certification. Relations would apply to a Justice of the Peace to have a disturbed member of the family admitted to Holywell. The patient would be taken by train by two policemen. Once certified, it was likely that the patient would remain in Holywell for some time, or indeed for ever. Patients in these early years of the hospital were controlled or cared for rather than treated.

One John Mayburn started at Holywell in 1942 and worked for thirty-nine years in the institution. He said that before the advent of the NHS it was a terrible place. Men were shaved once a week with one razor between many. Clothes were rough and shapeless. Men wore rough tweed suits, trousers often at half mast or rolled up, and their heads shorn. Women wore long black dresses up to their necks, and the clothes were made in the hospital. The sexes were strictly segregated, even at mealtimes. Meals were served in a large hall and only spoons were used to eat with. The diet appears to have been adequate: tea, bread and porridge for breakfast; beef, Irish stew or bacon for dinner, depending on the day (except for Fridays, when there was no meat but rice pudding was served); also there was tea and bread for tea. Tobacco was issued to those patients that were in work – the air in the corridors was full of smoke.

There were efforts to carry on a simple form of occupational therapy in Holywell. The recovery rate in these formative years was about forty-five per cent of admissions, but the hospital in October and November 1918 was caught up in a fever outbreak: 108 patients and staff fell ill, and seven patients died.

Smoking was regarded as a useful therapy for relaxation. This was an age in which drugs were unlikely to be used to treat conditions such as violent behaviour. Some of these unfortunate people needed to be restrained.

There was a marked effort on the part of the doctors to understand mental illness. Alcohol and hereditary causes explained many conditions. It was observed that many patients suffered from insanity that ran in families. In 1933 it was agreed to refer patients to Queen's University for examination and research.

There were few amusements for patients in the first decades of Holywell Hospital. In 1910, for example, patients walked daily in the grounds. The only other form of amusement appears to have been the weekly dance.

In 1923 the first overhaul of Holywell was undertaken. Spring Farm House was provided with a steam boiler which affected a large economy of fuel. The roof and walls were repaired; a sitting room was provided for the female, and later male, nursing staff.

In 1930, at about ten o'clock on 16 April, a fire broke out in the kitchen. Within minutes the flames had engulfed parts of the hospital, and the smoke could be seen as far away as Carrickfergus, fifteen miles distant. The fire brigade arrived from Belfast just as the roof of the Recreation Hall crashed in. Many people from Antrim town rushed up Steeple Road to help matters. A hundred gallons of tea were brewed and carried in buckets around the wards to the patients having their breakfast in bed. For months later the male patients dined in a large marquee which adjoined the main building. The cost of the fire damage was reckoned to be about £20,000, plus £160 for the cost of extinguishing the fire. But recovery from the fire was quite quick.

In February 1930 Dr Graham, the RMS, announced his intention to resign, and he was replaced by Dr Walter Smyth, but he died after six weeks of an illness in a Belfast nursing home. In appreciation of Dr Smyth it was agreed to place a portrait of him in Holywell's boardroom and a plaque was placed in the front hall, where it can still be seen.

CHAPTER THREE

NEW HORIZONS: 1932–47

The Mental Health Act was welcomed at Holywell in 1937. Voluntary patients now came into their own. It was said that early treatment for mental illness was essential. Certification was now a thing of the past upon admission. The word 'asylum' was dropped and replaced by 'mental hospital', and attendants became 'male nurses'. The new RMS brought fresh air into Holywell, for he wanted to involve the management committee more closely in the hospital's affairs.

Renovations were urgently needed at Holywell. Its broken ceilings, wards and corridors all needed repairs to bring things up to standard. The entire hospital was rewired with electric cables, and in 1933 work began on installing central heating. Under Dr Boyd's leadership the vermin problem was addressed for the first time in 1932, but rats continued to be a problem.

Boyd also attempted to inject energy into the social life of the patients and staff. Concerts and entertainments were given at intervals during the year. At Halloween the patients provided their own entertainment. A badminton court was also laid out in the Recreation Hall.

Female patients were now provided with light summer dresses. All patients, including the men, were provided with tweed outdoor coats.

Holywell's main building was at last provided with central heating, a new byre was built, and a new sewage plant installed. The year 1936 saw many improvements in Holywell, including a leisure garden.

The Bush House Estate was purchased in 1934 for £9,000; it was near to the main building, its grounds were fifty acres in extent, and there is a good view of Lough Neagh. When the house came on the market the intention was to use the house for private paying female patients. By the next year, 1935, Bush House had been completely overhauled, repaired and renovated. The house was tastefully and comfortably furnished. By 1942 there were thirty private patients resident at Bush House, each paying £3 3s. per week. Despite the purchase of Bush House, Dr Boyd was still concerned about overcrowding: Holywell was originally intended to hold 460 patients, and with the erection of the villa and the opening of Spring Farm House capacity had increased to 500. In 1934 the hospital population exceeded 600. Dr Boyd remarked in 1935 that overcrowding was the main problem. He recommended the extension of the existing buildings and the erection of a new admissions block. Extension blocks on the male and female sides of Holywell were completed in the summer of 1937.

In 1937 the staff and patients at Holywell were hit by its worst health crisis yet, for at the end of 1937 the hospital was the victim of an epidemic of colitis. Seventy-nine patients required isolation and a number of them died. The water supply was said to be the source of contamination. In 1938 there came an outbreak of paratyphoid B, and on 18 December two nurses and a female patient were transferred to the fever wards of the Massereene Hospital suffering from this disease. Twenty died. Help was called in from outside to deal with the crisis.

By 1938 there were 684 patients in Holywell – the greatest number ever. Now under the impact of the 1931 Mental Health Act, occupational therapy was introduced.

This was an attempt to involve patients in handicrafts and jobs under professional supervision. By 1933 twenty-five patients were benefiting. But in the late 1930s the initiative petered out. In the early 1930s the average cost per patient rose from £39 16s. 5d. in 1934 to £48 8s. 3d. This was due to economic factors. The situation was helped by increased receipts from paying patients, but by 1938 rising expenditure meant that a greater strain was put on these patients. In 1939 central-government grants to mental hospitals were increased by fifty per cent.

In the interwar years, conditions for the staff remained poor. The staff-to-patient ratio in 1939 was 1:72. In 1932 the RMS, Dr R. Boyd, warned the management committee that the hospital was understaffed, but four new male nursing posts, for which there were a number of applicants, were filled. At the time there were only three medical officers in Holywell for about 680 patients. Work was difficult for the new medical officers (i.e. doctors) before the Second World War, and there was no accommodation for visiting doctors. In 1930, fourteen members of the nursing staff at last began training for the certificate in mental nursing. The medical officers gave once-weekly lectures from October to May. All new medical staff were now expected to be qualified three years from the date of hiring. Those who received the certificate were granted a £2 10s. (five per cent) pay rise.

As with the First World War, inflation was at work in regards to wages. In 1940 the management committee conceded cash payments of only £5 yearly to all nursing staff and others in the hospital – for example, cooks and laundry maids. Wages in Holywell lagged behind those in England. In 1941 a central arbitration board for all mental hospitals in the UK effectively determined pay annually. Official TGWU meetings in hospitals (four per year) were permitted in 1946. On 18 April 1939, Dr Boyd died after a brief illness; he had served for seven years as RMS. Doctor Gilbert Smith took over in August, and he wished to make

Holywell a more attractive place for patients. He was in the job for twenty-seven years.

The Second World War meant that Holywell would have to comply with air-raid precautions, so blackout curtains were placed over the windows of the various rooms. In 1940 all patients were issued with gas masks, but the air-raid sirens disturbed them, causing many sleepless nights, and put extra burden on the staff. Some of the staff volunteered to fight in the war.

In 1940, with patients numbering about 680, it was agreed to build a new male and female admissions ward. The patients now came from Purdysburn at Belfast; a busload arrived with thirty patients and three nurses. By December, ninety-four patients (forty-four female and fifty male) had been transferred. This brought the total number of residents in Holywell from 680 in 1940 to 779, but this is spelled considerable overcrowding in the hospital. Rationing, difficulties in obtaining staff and the evacuating of patients had all added to the hospital's troubles. The war years were a harsh experience for the patients. To save on coal, patients were bathed once a fortnight rather than weekly, and clothes were changed frequently. The meals were improved with the addition of bacon one day per week. But the problem of infectious disease did not disappear, and during the war epidemics were quite common.

In 1940 there were a total of thirty cases – four male and twenty-six female. Acute cases of both colitis and dysentery were isolated in the upper dormitories of the chronic female wards, for the isolation wards were not large enough to accommodate all the patients who required to be isolated. Holywell lacked a good laundry where clothes could be adequately dealt with – especially very dirty garments.

In 1943, the clerk, Mr John Walker, the last veteran of Holywell's senior staff, decided to retire; the committee agreed to grant him a £200 bonus, for he was retiring for medical reasons. Walker died in 1949, aged eighty-five.

By working twelve years into his pension he had saved the taxpayer £2,000, but the committee disallowed the bonus. By the early 1940s the poor pay earned by medical staff made recruitment very difficult. Social life was restricted for the staff, particularly for the female side. In 1943 Dr Mary Robinson, the assistant medical officer, announced her intention to marry. The committee was unyielding: they agreed that they could not have a married female assistant on their payroll. The committee decided that it would be necessary to cancel her appointment, and Dr Robinson's marriage did not go ahead. In 1959 Dr Robinson reduced her working hours with sick notes to the hospital's authority. When the management committee protested she complained that her mail had been tampered with, and she refused to attend a disciplinary meeting on the grounds of family bereavement. Dr Robinson sought legal advice, but she did not win sick leave and her hours of work were reduced. She refused to cooperate and she was absent from work from 20 July to 27 September. Eventually she returned to work on the committee's terms, and no further action was taken against her.

During the war staff discontent was growing and maltreatment of patients was a developing problem. It was hoped that the recommendations of the Taylor Report on pay and conditions would attract a better sort of person to the service. Staff had to be in by ten o'clock at night. The doctors' rounds were cursory and patients were rarely talked to. Training in mental nursing was very limited, and it was based on a single book. There was one lecture on how to bandage, but otherwise lectures were single recitations from the textbook.

Recruitment was a problem at all staff levels, as the RMS reported in 1942.

In October 1944 the Rushcliffe Scheme came into effect in England, greatly improving social and work conditions for mental-hospital staff, and it was feared that staff might leave Holywell for better pay on the mainland, but there was a delay in fully introducing the proper scale of pay for mental nurses. Those nurses that remained in Holywell were becoming more dissatisfied with existing conditions.

Recruitment was still difficult after the war. The RMS reported in 1946 that a shortage of nurses due to sickness was making conditions difficult. As a stopgap, ex-servicemen were employed temporarily in the female mess room, but food was also a problem. Dormitory staff were also hard to find. During these years new forms of treatment had been introduced – notably, ECT (electroconvulsive therapy). A machine was bought for £54, replacing the hand-and-chain method. By November ECT was in service with good results. But ECT was at first a crude affair – one person dislocated her right shoulder during treatment, but she was able to return to Holywell the next day.

In 1943 a dental clinic opened and attempts were made to restart occupational therapy, two nurses (one male and one female) being sent for training in Britain. In 1946 an OT hut was opened and in 1949 a converted Spring Farm House was opened for OT.

Towards the end of the war discussions began on the opening of outpatient clinics to help treatment in the community. It was agreed that clinics should open at Ballymoney, Lisburn and Hillsborough District Hospitals. The first outpatient clinic opened in the Waveney Hospital in February 1947. It was followed by one in Larne and at Massereene in April, and afterwards in Ballymoney and Lisburn. By 1949 additional staff had been found. Dr Smith reported in 1950 that a large number of outpatients were suffering with nervous disorders, and that the treatment would take time.

Shortly after the war Holywell was in dire straits. A committee recommended the appointment of a resident engineer to control building, joinery and repair work and to coordinate the staff in such activities.

After the Second World War a musical band was formed to entertain the patients on a weekly basis. A new tuck shop was opened so that patients could buy what they wanted with money supplied by relatives. Tokens were supplied by the hospital. New roads were laid in the grounds, an OT centre was built, new laundry equipment was provided and a cinema was installed. Attempts were made to improve the quality of the food – there was now more variety on the menu – and a staff restaurant was also opened, but it was still hard to find a manager for the kitchen. As previously mentioned, new wooden huts were used for OT. By 1949 much had been achieved; the old idea of the lunatic asylum had been shelved. Now came the National Health Service, and Holywell was poised to play a role.

CHAPTER FOUR

A NATIONAL HEALTH SERVICE
HOSPITAL

After the Second World War, in 1946 the National Health Service Act was passed, and from then on money continued to flow into the NHS. Holywell was a beneficiary. A new hospital authority had come into existence, but Bush House would continue to be a private adjunct. The new name for the asylum was to be Holywell Hospital. The RMS advocated an admissions/convalescent unit to house about 130 patients, but overcrowding in the hospital resulted in 139 patients, both male and female. The stigma of mental illness was now set aside in these liberal years (1949–2018), and an increasing number of patients came forward for treatment to the outpatient clinic. The Tobervaneen units were now constructed, Tobervaneen being the Irish for Holywell. They were officially opened on 15 November 1954 by the Minister of Health and Social Services. But there were internal problems, including dampness that affected the walls, floors and furniture.

Financial restraints eased in the 1950s, so Holywell embarked on a number of improvements and modifications to the hospital, including the refitting of the hospital's kitchen. Patients now went to bed later instead of at eight o'clock in the evening. Patients could go on holiday – especially long-stay patients.

Treatment for the criminally insane had not improved.

The admissions rate of voluntary patients had at first not been much affected, but by 1968 there was no provision for highly disturbed patients in Northern Ireland, this being left for the 2000s. There was now more interaction with patients in the local Antrim community. Local dances attracted many people from a wide area. In 1950 Massereene Hospital in Antrim established a psychiatry unit complete with beds. Holywell itself developed an aftercare service for discharged patients. Patients were now visited in their own homes by a social worker, and people were referred to outpatient departments. OT now came into its own. The present OT department, based at the villa, is one of the most advanced in the UK.

In 1956 plans were put forward to expand Holywell to take patients from Purdysburn Hospital, Belfast. Inpatient numbers would now rise to over 1,000. In 1961 a major new mental health Act was passed by the Stormont government, which would change policies and attitudes to mental health. Now patients would be admitted and discharged in the same way as at other general hospitals. The Act also affected those patients living in the community. Communal care was the objective. The treatment of older people was now addressed, but the wards were still overcrowded and patients also lacked privacy. Some films were produced about Holywell.

In 1955 Holywell began to consider the possibility of establishing a day hospital in Belfast; this would be the first day hospital in Northern Ireland. Patients would be treated on an outpatient basis. Suitable patients for inclusion in the scheme were those suffering from schizophrenia and depressive disorders. Of the 214 patients admitted to Holywell during the first three months in 1959, it was found that eighty-two could have been treated at a day hospital, and about half of these would not need inpatient treatment at any stage. Accommodation remained an acute problem during 1959. Senior staff at Holywell oversaw some sixty-seven male and seventy-eight female staff. Pressures were acute on the female side.

Holywell was also a training hospital, and movements to improve standards became marred in the late 1960s. With the increase of admissions, Holywell's clerical staff came under pressure. It was proposed that nurses should be allowed to sleep out and that sleeping-in would be on a rota basis. There was an effort to have staff involved in the running of the hospital.

The late 1950s saw the introduction of drawing therapy, a revolutionary step for those suffering from depression and other illnesses, to perhaps shorten their stay in hospital. By the 1960s patients were encouraged to wear their own clothes rather than a uniform. They were given thirteen shillings pocket money per week if they had no other income. Those working obtained thirty-five shillings per week.

Dr Smith retired due to ill health in 1967. As a result of his policies there were 993 admissions and 982 discharges. There were a total of 3,232 outpatients visited. Staff numbers over a long period had reached 444.

Spring Farm, since its opening, was an important source of food produce for the patients and staff. Work on the farm was meant to be therapeutic in the treatment of insanity. The purchase of Bush House in 1934 increased the size of the farm to 154 acres. The farm was organized for OT purposes and not for commercial gain. By the late 1960s the farm provided occupations for forty patients. Spring Farm finally closed on 31 March 1971. Industrial therapy would take its place. In 1970 an industrial Advisory Office was established – 150 patients would receive training. But the care for patients still left much to be desired, for pharmacy and dispensary services were substandard, and there was a shortage of beds.

The medical superintendent of the hospital was now Dr Enda Casement, who had replaced Dr Smith.

The Northern Ireland Troubles had little effect on the hospital, but all inter-hospital activities were suspended, to be resumed in 1972. At Holywell there were bomb alerts. Shortly after his retirement in 1984, at the age of sixty-two, Dr Casement's house was the scene of a bomb alert. By the end of Dr Casement's career the medical staff at Holywell was greatly increased. The drift was now towards shorter periods of admission; also segregation between male and female patients was ended. Integration of staff became obligatory only in 1985. In an effort to end long-term admissions, patients were encouraged to return to society. In 1972 the social workers in Holywell were increased. In 1966 a hostel with six beds was opened in Ballymena. A hostel at Holywell was opened in 1970 to help long-stay patients. In 1971 other hostels were opened at Rathfern, Newtownabbey, Gurten and Longview. In 1985 Bush House became a rehabilitation unit, where long-term patients were encouraged to return to the community. In 1991 a patient carer unit was established – the first of its kind in Northern Ireland.

Dr David King succeeded Dr Casement in 1993. He had developed the theory that mental illness, especially mood disorders, are caused by a chemical imbalance in the brain; and he introduced drugs like clozapine to help matters. After a year at Purdysburn he went to Sheffield; now he became confirmed in his view that mental illnesses are due to a chemical imbalance in the brain. He returned to Belfast to study neurology. He worked for three years at the Medical Research Foundation, in London, where he was given an MD. He returned to Holywell in 1972 at the age of thirty-one. He continued his research into mood disorders. Now he introduced lithium to help in the treatment of manic depressive disorders – the first lithium clinic of its kind in Northern Ireland.

After eighteen months Dr King came went to Canada as assistant professor to Bob Jones at Dalhousie University, but he was invited to return to Ulster to take up the post of senior lecturer in clinical neuropharmacology at Queen's University and at Holywell. He took up the joint post in October 1975. The death of one of Holywell's female patients had revealed unsatisfactory practice in drug dispensing, but pharmacy research was improved. Dr King now took over two locked wards – one male and the other female – for highly disturbed patients. New drugs are coming on to the market all the time. Clinical studies, such as an investigation of the possibility that viruses cause mental illness, were also carried out in Holywell. Dr King pursued a programme of drug trials in the hospital, focusing on schizophrenia, and the use of drugs like clozapine since the 1970s, and there were few side effects. Dr King believed that enlightened attitudes to mental illness were only possible because of advances in drug treatment. Dr Freeman held the opposite view – that mental illness is emotionally produced – but the two men got on well together. Innovations continued with the use of medication for serious disorders, like the dementias. Dr King continued his close association with Queen's University, Belfast. He lectured at Queen's, where he became a professor, as well as writing a number of papers and chapters in books, and editing textbooks for the Royal College of Physicians. Holywell's research centre has helped to put Northern Ireland on the map as far as the treatment of mental illness is concerned. Holywell has become a favourite training hospital for medical studies.

In the care of the very disturbed in locked wards, policy changes were due to the introduction of new drugs and the use of ECT (electric-shock treatment). Now new drugs have meant that the patient may return to the community or to an exit ward and is able to receive help at the various outpatient clinics. In the ten years from 1958 expenditure on drugs increased by 100 per cent. The villa has changed from a ward to the OT centre. Professor King was Holywell's medical superintendent and chairman of the medical staff from 1993 to 1996. A five-year plan to reduce hospital beds by over one-third, from 500 to 325, was announced in 1992, and it was promised that no jobs would be lost. Long-term beds were to be reduced from eighty-five to thirty-six, and other beds from 165 to 110; other units came into existence in Ballymena, Moyle and Coleraine. Holywell remains the acute centre for Antrim, Ballymena, Magherafelt and Cookstown.

Holywell now has 108 acute admissions beds in the three Tobervaneen units. There is now a day hospital. Professor King will be remembered for his pioneering of modern drugs and his help in changing the attitude of society to mental illness.